P9-EIG-742

How to Steal from a Medical Practice

Guide to embezzling and how to prevent it

By

Donald R. Elton, MD, FCCP

Donald R. Elton

ISBN-13: 978-1456593629

ISBN-10: 1456593625

Copyright © 2011 by Donald R. Elton - All Rights Reserved

Dedication

This book is dedicated to all of my honest and hardworking employees over the years. To the others? Not so much.

Warning

This book is not a substitute for professional advice from your attorney or your accountant. Nothing contained in this text should be construed as professional legal or accounting advice. Any suggestions made are solely the opinion of the author and should be verified with professional counsel prior to implementation in your business.

Table of Contents

Part I - Best practices

Introduction

Embezzlement from medical practices is very common. A Google search of "Medical Embezzlement" yields over 700,000 hits. Consider the following recent news excerpts:

> She started by keeping some of the cash from the co-payments for herself and altering information in the computer to make it look as if it was an insurance write-off. "It got to the point where she was not recording any cash she received from these doctors' offices."

> A former medical worker pleaded not guilty Tuesday to stealing over $100,000 from her former employer. Sixty-two-year-old Ann BlahBlah worked as an office

worker at BlahBlah Family Physicians for more than 10 years. Police say she stole the money by altering paperwork to cover her actions.

Police on Thursday charged a woman with stealing almost $200,000 from a medical practice. Janet SorryThief, was charged with embezzlement greater than $100,000. She was being held in the County Jail under a $50,000 bond. A physician with the practice asked police last month to investigate money missing from the practice. Investigators determined SorryThief used business credit cards and checks to amass nearly $200,000 in purchases over a 5 year period. SorryThief was the business manager for the practice until she was fired in October, police said.

The unfortunate fact is that you really don't know as much about your employees as you think you do. This is particularly true when you first hire someone. Even if you hire an all-star employee whose references and criminal background you've checked, you never really know who may change from a trusted employee into one who steals from your practice perhaps due to changes in their personal circumstance. A desperate need for extra money coupled with an easy opportunity to steal is a temptation that many will find difficult to resist. This doesn't mean that checking out prospective employees is a waste of time. When you are hiring someone who will work in the reception area or billing office or management you need to be particularly careful and make a good effort to avoid hiring people who already have a criminal background. There are many

online sources for background information such as

http://www.ussearch.com,

http://www.intellius.com,

and many other sites. The services are typically not free

but neither are the results of hiring an employee with a

criminal background to handle your cash flow.

http://www.oig.hhs.gov/fraud/exclusions.asp

This site lets you check to see if a potential employee (or

even physician) has been banned from participation in

Medicare or Medicaid activities due to fraud.

The sites won't find everyone who has been caught stealing as only 29% of employees caught stealing from their medical practice employer get prosecuted. Therefore, the majority of those caught will not have a record and who can say how many are stealing still and just haven't been caught yet, much less prosecuted? These sorts of search sites can show information about property owned, criminal convictions, sex offender registries, prior addresses, and more. A Google search (http://www.google.com) and searches of Facebook (http://www.facebook.com), MySpace (http://www.myspace.com), LinkedIn (http://www.linkedin.com, Twitter (http://www.twitter.com), and other social media sites can reveal information about potential hires (and existing employees) that may tip you off to lifestyles more extravagant than their legitimate income can support.

Reviewing prior work history and looking for jobs left off the CV can be telling. It has been more difficult in recent years to find prior employers who are willing to give a bad reference about a former employee to a stranger. A clue may be a reference unwilling to give out more than dates of hire and termination - employers are more likely to be forthcoming when the information to be passed on is positive. It may help to have the potential employee sign a consent granting permission to all prior employers to give out truthful information on their work history but many prior employers will still be too afraid of potential liability to give you useful negative information. Sometimes Google is your best friend. We've had applicants provide a

CV with all sorts of work experience and a five minute Google search showed evidence of current or former employment that was not listed on the CV. Even though this omission may not mean this person was a thief it does tell you they don't have any problem with dishonesty. When combined with need and opportunity, dishonesty is not something you really want in a new hire.

You may want to consider having key employees such as your manager or billing department staff bonded. Bonding is a process where an insurer investigates the employees' background and then issues a special insurance policy that covers you in the event that the bonded employee steals from you. See http://www.demerittagency.com/ bonding_your_business.pdf for more information on bonding and how you can use bonding in your business.

An employee can steal from your practice in many ways, and this book is not exhaustive as criminals continue to create new ways to take your property. I've been on the receiving end of some of the methods described here and you should know that if an employee starts stealing using one method, he or she is likely to employ other methods depending on the opportunities you either provide or that the employee thinks you are providing. Not all employee theft can or will be prevented. You should not be so confident in your abilities to prevent or detect theft that you have your overconfidence taken advantage of. You should also prepare for theft that may be occurring or that may occur in the future to minimize the damage done to your business financially and otherwise. For most of us who own and operate a small business, an employee in a trusted position who steals from us is a very personal and disturbing thing. Being a victim makes us question how we could have been fooled into trusting someone unworthy and creates a strong feeling of wanting the perpetrator punished both as a form of retribution and justice and to set an example to other employees who might someday be tempted. Unfortunately, employee theft may not be a priority of the legal system in your area so do not count on the police being eager to send anyone to jail. It is to be hoped that the methods described in this book will help you recognize and manage your vulnerabilities and help you prepare to limit your losses should theft occur.

How common is employee theft? The Medical Group Management Association

http://www.mgma.com released a survey in 2010 reporting that 83% of practice managers had been with a medical practice at some point that had experienced employee theft. The MGMA survey also said that nearly 20% of incidents involved losses of $100,000 or more. The MGMA survey estimated that only 29% of embezzlers were prosecuted and only 83% were terminated from their jobs. This is amazing to me that 17% of embezzlers from medical practices not only were probably not prosecuted, they didn't even lose their jobs after being caught.

Why is embezzlement from medical practices so common? Famous bank robber Willie Sutton was instructive:

"Why did I rob banks? Because I enjoyed it. I loved it. I was more alive when I was inside a bank, robbing it, than at any other time in my life. I enjoyed everything about it so much that one or two weeks later I'd be out looking for the next job. But to me the money was the chips, that's all." "Go where the money is...and go there often." [Where the Money Was: The Memoirs of a Bank Robber (Viking Press, New York, 1976)]

Why do employees steal from medical practices? Many reasons. The thrill described by Mr. Sutton may be one of the factors keeping an employee going back to the habit. Other elements include:

Financial need

Divorce

Gambling

Substance abuse

Need to pay for an affair

Spousal job loss

Personal or Family illness

To prove they're smarter than employer

Trying to get the pay they "deserve"

Getting even with employer

Doctors are rich and won't miss it anyway

The overwhelming reason though why theft from medical practices is so common is that it's so easy to do and so easy to get away with it.

Physicians typically don't realize how common and expensive employee theft is. As a result we don't consider the possibility very often and tend to trust our staff more than we should. Not only do we tend to not look for vulnerabilities or create internal controls to make employee theft difficult, we are also slow to notice it when it happens and many times don't even consider the possibility until we are ourselves running short of funds. Once detected we can't believe it happened. We are embarrassed we let it happen. We are angry at the perpetrators or maybe others we think should have prevented the theft. We are typically very hurt that someone in a position of trust did this to us. After the initial shock and anger passes, many practices just want to keep the whole thing quiet and move on which may

account for why only one-third of employee thieves ever

have charges pressed against them. When you decide you

want to press charges to punish the perpetrator and as a

deterrent to others who might consider stealing from you,

you may find your local police or sheriff's departments

don't take the crime nearly as seriously as you do, and are

likely to work hard to find a way to avoid having the

criminal serve time in jail. All of this makes it increasingly

difficult to protect your practice when the whole system

seems to encourage theft at every level.

The thieves usually know a lot more about how to steal

and cover their crimes than their employers know about

how to deter, prevent, detect, and punish these criminals.

Even when you fire someone who steals from you, odds are good they will stay in the medical field and move to another practice where they can take advantage of even more physicians who haven't read this book yet.

A recent article in American Medical News estimated that 10% of employees will never steal, 10% will always steal, and 80% will steal if given the opportunity. The truth is, if you stay in the practice of medicine long enough it's only a matter of time until you are a victim of employees stealing from you.

Prepare for theft

Every year more and more small businesses are damaged by fraud and embezzlement. The Association of Certified Fraud Examiners http://www.acfe.com/ reported that small businesses in the United States lose about half a trillion dollars per year and that nearly half of all workplace fraud occurs in small businesses. The risk is especially high in medical practices, particularly those that are privately owned and small. Think about it, how much training did you get in medical school about how to prevent theft by employees? Most of us have no business training or experience of any kind when we finish our medical training. Few of us are able to hire people who have the sort of training we really need. If we're financially able to hire the caliber of people we really need, how many of us know what to look for or how to even know if the person we hire to protect us is going to be the next thief?

The worst thing you can do running a medical practice is to assume that your employees are all trustworthy and that employee theft cannot or will not happen to you. This overconfidence is not only a perfect setup for the employee who wants to steal from you, it also prevents you from doing what you need to do in advance to make it more likely you will prevent, detect, and be able to recover from theft.

Balance

No practice is 100% safe from theft. You can think about every method presented in this text and employ every safeguard but eventually someone will find or create a hole in your security. A practice, bank, or even nuclear power plant with 100% effective security is by its nature nonfunctional. You have to strike a balance between keeping your practice secure from foreseeable and likely risks and keeping the work environment productive for you and your staff. You probably don't leave your wallet on the table at a restaurant when you go to the rest room and you shouldn't leave cash unattended in your office either. You could hire an armed guard to follow all of your employees and could require invasive searches of everyone who enters or leaves your building every time, but who would guard the guards and how would any work get done and who would pay for all this? Taking reasonable common sense precautions will prevent most theft and allow you to detect most of what slips by you but there comes a point when insurance is cheaper and more effective than creating more security than your potential losses may justify. In this book I try to present information on the typical and common threats to a practice so you can understand most of the methods thieves use to steal from their medical practice employers. Armed with this information you can implement reasonable internal controls and auditing methods to deter and detect theft. Additional information is presented to help you recover from theft after the fact should it occur in spite of your efforts to deter it.

Don't concentrate

Avoid concentrating too much responsibility with any one person. If you have one person working check-in, check-out, billing, opening mail, and paying bills, you are asking for trouble on multiple levels. Not only have you made it easy for such a person to steal from you with little oversight or accountability, you have also made your practice highly dependent on one individual who will be difficult to replace. If your "key employee" should happen to quit or get sick or injured you can really have problems if no one else is trained to handle their duties.

Separate critical duties among several staffers and cross-train them to be able to perform at least one other job in your practice so that one employee's departure will not cripple your practice. Dividing responsibility is more difficult in a small practice with only a few employees though cross training becomes even more important as a single employee's illness or vacation causes a much larger problem for the small practice than for a big one. When the practice is small, it's likely that you will be best off with one or more practice owners taking over key parts of the cash flow process such as opening the mail to remove any payments before the mail goes anywhere else. If you can't manage to have an owner do all the mailbox runs then set a policy forbidding anyone other than an owner or a person in an owners presence from opening bank and credit card statements. It's important to make sure no one can remove pages of statements or copies of checks to hide fraudulent transactions. This policy will not, however, keep someone from just intentionally losing the entire statement from time to time so I still believe it is best for a practice owner to keep the mailbox keys and to open or personally supervise the opening of all incoming mail. The owners need to be involved in setting up processes to prevent and deter and detect theft and need to be closely involved in at least weekly if not daily reconciliation of collections that occur at the office. If you follow the advice given later about keeping money away from the office by way of direct wired payments from insurers and use of a Lockbox then the amount of cash that needs to be tracked and that is available for theft at the office can be greatly limited.

Team players

We all talk about how we want our employees to be good team players. However, too much teamwork can be a liability. Just as it's important to avoid concentrating too many responsibilities in any single employee, you need to pay attention to friendships and alliances among your staff that create a situation where two or more staffers can team up to steal from you. Such teams may be created when you hire a close friend of an existing employee, when employees meet after you hire them and become close friends or lovers, or when you hire family members of existing employees. In some cases the "team" will indeed be a premeditated criminal conspiracy that will plot for ways to steal. In other cases, one "team member" will take advantage of the loyalty of the other player and will do the stealing betting that their "partner" will look the other way

or will in some other way facilitate the theft. What can you

do about this? You can't really prevent employees from

becoming friends either on the job or off the job but in

cases where you have split duties such as creating the

deposit slip and taking the deposit to the bank you have to

make sure you aren't really using two people who

effectively function as one for this duty. This defeats the

purpose of avoiding the "concentration" mentioned in the

prior chapter. If you decide to separate ordering supplies

from the person who takes inventory and distributes what

is delivered, then again you have to avoid assigning this to

a team. In a small practice with few employees, these sorts

of teams or alliances are more difficult to work around as

you may not have many alternatives other than to use a

team member from time to time but you do need to be

aware of the risk and be particularly vigilant when you are

forced to do this.

'Tis the season

Be particularly alert for theft from about December 1 until about February 15. Why? Two reasons. One is that the Christmas gift giving season is a time when many people will look for supplemental income. Two, most patients with insurance have their deductibles reset between December 1 and January 1. This means there will hopefully be an increase in patient payments for their visits during December and January as their insurers will not be paying until those patients meet their deductible. With so many people now having high deductible insurance plans, there will be many patients who will never meet their deductible thus they'll be required to pay more of their bill to the practice. Combine necessity with opportunity and one can expect there will be more theft of patient payments during this part of the year.

Most practices see a drop in cash flow every year during the period when no one's deductible has been met. This means that theft occurring during this time will have more potential to do harm to the fiscal health of your practice.

Embezzler characteristics

How do you recognize an embezzler or potential embezzler? Some are your more intelligent employees who may not feel appreciated for their knowledge or skills. Thieves run the spectrum though - some are not so smart and will do stupid things that get them caught quickly. The smarter employees are really more of a threat just as the longtime trusted employees are more of a threat. Here are some other things to look for:

Someone stealing from you may be reluctant to have other people do their duties and may be slow to train others to cover for their duties. They may avoid taking vacation time for fear someone else in their position even temporarily may see irregularities. When they are away from the office they may feel they are losing the opportunity to steal. A company policy that requires employees to take at least one vacation of at least 3 contiguous days per year may be helpful.

You may notice that someone in your employ is taking more expensive vacations than usual or buying items someone in their position would not normally be able to afford. The most common characteristic of an embezzler? They are frequently long time loyal trusted employees that you would never dream would be stealing from their employer. Employee theft usually starts almost innocently with "borrowing" from petty cash or practice credit cards, manipulating time clock times to get more paid hours, or appropriating pens or printer supplies. Once they get away with the small stuff it can either be fun or profitable or

good for their ego since they get the idea they're smarter

than their bosses and deserve the extra income they're able

to walk away with. Some look at theft as a way to pay

back an employer they perceive as making too much

money or not appreciating their loyalty. There are

hundreds of ways for criminals to rationalize criminal

behavior but the truth is that they are criminals and crime

is what criminals do.

Know what you have

Your medical practice business has many things of value. You need to know what you have that others may covet and steal before you can devise strategies to protect your valuables or to recover in the event some of your valuables are taken. Here are some categories of valuables or potential areas of losses for most practices:

Tangible

Computers, computer peripherals, computer software, furniture, art, medications, samples, test equipment, lab equipment, microscopes, televisions, tools, paper supplies, printer ink and toner.

Financial

Cash, incoming checks, outgoing checks, credit cards and debit cards

Indirect or intangible

Bribes & kickbacks, referrals (incoming and outgoing), theft of time (on the clock), patient information, business information

Employer liability for employee crime

Drug diversion, insurance fraud, patient confidentiality, sexual harassment claims, worker's compensation claims, discrimination charges (race, sex, disability)

Take inventory of what you have

You should maintain an inventory both video and written of all the tangible assets you have. You need this so you can tell when things are missing (which of course means you have to regularly and perhaps randomly check on items from your written inventory sheet to make sure you still have the items in your possession). You also need this to help with an insurance claim should one be needed. Be sure to keep track of the value of each item on your inventory both for the police and your insurer. Make sure you keep a copy of the inventory offsite where an office fire or other disaster can't destroy it. Make sure you have sufficient insurance to cover the replacement cost of all the important items from your list. Note that replacement cost is different from and usually more than actual current value for most items. Talk to your insurer about this.

Consider getting insurance to cover for loss of income

while you are closed and rebuilding if you really suffer a

big or important (say your medical records or billing

databases) loss.

Monitor / protect

You have to monitor your valuables and make visible efforts to protect your valuables. Limit access to expensive items to those who must have access to do their jobs. Restrict access outside of normal business hours and limiting access to computers (business, medical records, and medical billing) to locations where employees can be supervised and know they are supervised. Lock doors and cabinets. Consider video, audio, and computer monitoring to deter, detect, and should theft or fraud occur to help build a case against the correct responsible parties for use in prosecution. Monitor employee business email accounts. If you don't know how to set it up, ask your internet service provider how you can archive and save at least several weeks of everyone's incoming and outgoing email.

This way if you discover or suspect something, you can go back and read emails from weeks prior that may uncover what is going on. Once an employee figures out you suspect them it's not very likely they will continue to write incriminating emails though I have seen it happen before. You can also install key logging software on any computer you own.

See http://www.spectorsoft.com

These programs are inexpensive and can record everything viewed or typed on the computer including web sites visited, passwords entered, mail or instant messages, and so on. The software can even look for specific words to be typed and email you an image of whatever was on the screen at the time the offending words are typed.

Monitored alarm systems should be not only installed but should be used. Individual disarm codes for anyone who may be the first to arrive or last to leave can allow you to monitor who enters the office and when. Employees must know that password sharing is a termination level offense and that they are personally responsible for anything that happens when they are logged in whether they were present or not. Employees can be required to sign a computer security policy when they are hired (or even later) that acknowledges that they accept full responsibility for anything that happens when they are logged into a computer in your office. The policy should further specify that they will be both legally and financially responsible.

If a credit card purchase must be made for the practice by anyone other than a business owner, then you can obtain a disposable credit card number for that purpose (i.e. one time use) so that the card information cannot be used later for nonbusiness fraudulent purchases.

You must have a system in place that splits duties in a way that employees are put in a position of helping you monitor the activities of others. You as the business owner, have to be involved in the business of the practice whether you like it or not. This means personally reviewing and sometimes balancing checking accounts, credit card statements, and monthly bills.

If appropriate require two signatures for all business checks. Do not allow wire transfers or automatic bill pay either by way of a web site or office accounting software such as Quickbooks (TM) as these bypass the requirement for signatures to transmit money from your account.

Future chapters will examine some of these threats in more detail. It is critical that you not only know what you have, but that you watch what you have, and that everyone who may be tempted to steal knows you are indeed watching and paying attention. Being busy will be a weak excuse after you've been a victim of fraud.

Lockbox service

The Lockbox is when you have a PO box to which all patient payments and insurance payments are mailed. This keeps the money and the checks out of your office. This is best used with a bank that offers a Lockbox Service. This means the bank goes and checks your PO box every day using a bonded insured employee. They take the contents of the lockbox and open everything that looks like a payment. Checks and cash are copied and deposited directly into your bank account and the remaining box contents (mail, EOB's, copies of checks and cash and so on) are then either mailed to, delivered to, or picked up by your office minus the money that is already in your bank account. At that point your staff can use the returned material to post the payments, adjustments, and so on into the billing system and the actual payments are never in the office to tempt anyone with sticky fingers. The lockbox additionally is convenient if you change office locations as your pay-to address never changes. While the lockbox method is very helpful, you should know that not every bank offers the service and the service usually has a small cost associated with it. Even though all the statements will list this PO box as the pay-to address, there will still be some patients who will continue to mail their material straight to the office. This requires, as noted earlier, that an owner or manager control access to the mailbox so that any monies received are separated from the mail before it is passed off to anyone else. If an owner isn't getting the mail it may be best to require that two employees retrieve and open the mail to discourage one of them from diverting incoming items improperly. In a multiple doctor

practice it is best if this duty is rotated among doctors.

First it spreads the work around but it also allows the

doctor-partners to keep an eye on each other and allows

each to become familiar with and invested in fraud

prevention and detection.

Most major insurers will direct deposit their payments into

your practice account if you ask them to. As of this writing

our practice gets direct wired payments from Medicare,

Medicaid, the various Blue Cross insurers, United

Healthcare, Cigna, and several others. It's now actually

rare to receive insurance checks directly to the office. We

are also setup to receive insurer Explanation of Benefits

(EOB's) electronically that in many cases are

automatically posted to patient accounts. All of this apart from saving time and effort on the part of our billing staff keeps this money away from the office and away from anyone who might be inclined to divert incoming income to the practice. All practices should consider these options when available.

Computer security

Whole books are written on this topic. Medical practices use computers for billing, medical records, financial transactions, payroll, and communications. Many times the same computers are used for all of these functions. Add to this employees using their workstations to access Facebook, IM accounts, email (personal and business) and to download the latest video or porn site and every computer on the network becomes a potential site of invasion and compromise of your network. Not only do you risk losing valuable financial information you risk giving up your passwords and account numbers and just letting a hacker clean you out because an employee opened an email attachment sent to him or her and opened at work. In my experience, no matter how much you warn employees or even doctors about these risks, viruses still wind up taking over office computers from time to time and create lost time and headaches at best and a business closing disaster is always a potential risk.

At a minimum, every business (and home) computer network needs a hardware firewall installed and properly configured. If you don't know how to do this then hire someone big enough you have the legitimate option to sue them and hold them financially liable if they do it incorrectly. You need virus protection on every computer and up to date with automatic scanning and system protection 24/7. There are some free options available but paid options are more likely to be kept up to date and to not contain Trojan horse features themselves. The better packages help monitor your entire network and can email or text message you if any computer on your network becomes infected.

Your firewall needs to block access to websites that are more likely to be used for nonbusiness purposes than for business purposes. This would include but is not limited to facebook.com, match.com, plentyoffish.com chemistry.com, myspace.com, cupid.com, and many others you can probably think of. (If you're not sure, just ask your kids.) A good firewall will also keep logs that list every site accessed by every computer on your network. This will give you more information on where people may be wasting your paid time and give you names of other sites worth blocking. Firewalls capable of blocking porn sites are a good idea as these sites are notorious sources of malware. You can also set your server's network policies to restrict the downloading of attachments in email and various other options depending upon your risk tolerance and need for free communication.

You need to have reliable and tested backup strategies for critical computers on your network and if possible keep offline backups offsite. If your data size and network speed is not sufficient to automate this by way of the internet then you can buy a few portable USB drives and rotate them once a week putting a copy at home while the other is in the office collecting current backups. Keep at least a weeks worth of backups as some corruption issues wind up in all your backups if you don't discover a problem until a week after it appeared.

As for the employees, you can limit personal online transactions to a certain extent by reminding them that you have and regularly use your legal access to everything that goes on with your network including but not limited to reading their email and recording any passwords they enter on your systems. Once they know and are regularly reminded that they have no expectation of privacy for anything they do using your telephones and computers they'll be less likely to conduct personal business using your hardware while you're paying them for work they should have been doing instead of stealing time and endangering your data.

It is critical for security and for your legal responsibility for the veracity of medical record entries that passwords never be shared and that employees never use another person's login to do anything on the computer. The password is basically your's and your employee's electronic signature. If you're going to swear to the accuracy of an electronic medical record entry in a court case someday (and eventually you will) you will have to accept, as will your employees, responsibility for any entry made using your password even if it wasn't you that made the entry. This is really critical and it's not an easy task to make employees really believe this. It may take firing someone for a violation of this policy for the rest to take it seriously. As mentioned earlier, all employees should be required to sign a statement acknowledging that they are responsible for their passwords and anything that happens

using their password including but not limited to financial

responsibility.

Part II - General theft and fraud

Theft through incompetence

This chapter is about financial losses due to incompetence. This can be as simple as a biller choosing to never follow-up on claims that haven't been paid or as involved as a manager failing to supervise and detect substandard billing work on the part of an employee or worse yet seeing the work is of poor quality and doing nothing to either correct the behavior or terminate the employee. While many employees are truly loyal and grateful for the opportunities they've been given, there are others who have no interest in your business concerns so long as they get paid on time. Your practice loses money when you have staff that don't care enough about the financial health of your business to make sure all your services are charged for and paid for. It seems obvious perhaps to the business owner that all of these things matter but unfortunately, the financial health of your practice will typically not matter that much to your staff unless or until you fail to pay a payroll on time or otherwise have a situation such as a pay cut or benefit cut that affects them. Even when times are tough, you're as likely as not to be blamed for a situation that perhaps was at least partially their fault. That said, don't be too hard on them - they just work there. You are the one who hired them and presumably trained them to work the way they do whether intentionally or not. You, as the business owner, are ultimately responsible for supervising your staff including supervising your manager. You have a right to expect your employees to do their jobs properly, but it's up to you to correct the situation if they don't.

If you demonstrate to your staff that you aren't concerned about waste then don't expect them to be very concerned. If you make arbitrary or wasteful purchases of equipment or supplies, don't be surprised if your staff follows your lead. If you borrow money from the petty cash fund don't be surprised if your employees follow your lead. If you don't keep track of inventory or make sure you use the best vendors, then why would you expect your staff to behave otherwise? If you don't get personally involved in your medical billing and collection process, don't be surprised if your staff gets sloppy or lazy or indeed tempted to just steal from you emboldened by your complacency. This may be redundant but it's just as important to look interested as it is to be interested. Employees need to see and understand that you care about efficiency and avoiding fraud and your actions speak louder than your words in this regard.

Avoiding "theft" through incompetence starts with the hiring decision. Unfortunately it's impossible to avoid hiring someone who is not competent from time to time. You can improve your odds by checking references but not many employees will give you references that they expect to give you bad reviews of their work habits. Many employers are afraid to tell the truth even when they know the limitations of a former employee. Because you will likely hire some incompetent staff from time to time it's important that you constantly evaluate what you have. Set goals of what they should be able to do and by when. If they aren't meeting the goals in the agreed upon time, and if you don't see something you can fix, then you're better off replacing the employee rather than wasting more money trying to "train up" someone who just doesn't have the skills or attitude needed to get done what you need done. While training a new employee is expensive, a bad manager or bad biller (i.e. incompetent) will cost you more than most thieves could dream of taking from you.

Hiring a medical biller in a small practice that will only have one person doing the billing is a challenge. Many people who will answer an advertisement for such a position may have very little if any medical billing experience; those applicants aren't too difficult to detect.

More difficult though is that some people have worked one or more billing related positions, or positions that included some billing work yet have never been in a position of having to work every billing position. When you have a position for someone doing all of medical billing, particularly when others in the practice have little if any experience with medical billing, you are really looking for someone who can do charge entry, insurance filing, electronic and paper claims, patient payment posting, insurance payment, adjustment, and denial posting, collection calls to patients, insurance claim status checks, clearinghouse setup and trouble shooting, and more. The regulatory environment and insurance industry are constantly changing and you, as the physician are responsible for thousands of pages of billing related regulations even if you are just an employee and not the owner of the practice. You not only risk not getting paid; you can be required to pay back hundreds of thousands of dollars of money previously paid by insurers or Medicare and can be banned from future participation with those payers if they determine your billing was fraudulent even if it was just an incompetent biller who was doing the bad things. People who have worked medical billing in a large practice or hospital setting in most cases will not have the experience to do all of these things unless they were the billing manager and maybe not even then. It's obviously difficult to hire someone to do something you are not yourself qualified to perform or adequately supervise beyond seeing if you get a paycheck. The owner and/or the practice manager, even if not involved in day to day regular billing duties, must make it a point to learn both the entire billing process as well as learn how to use and monitor the use of the billing software. By the time an inadequate biller causes cash flow problems it's already much later you think; the mess created by a bad biller can take months to repair. Remember that some insurers will not pay for any claims filed beyond 90 days from the date of service so some money will be lost forever.

Theft of supplies

Theft and diversion of supplies that you use in your practice can include everything from soda's and snacks for the break room to pens, paper, forms, toner and ink cartridges, toilet paper, paper towels, and more. This can also include medical supplies such as medications, IV start materials, needles, and syringes, and various other items that are used and disposed of and reordered from time to time.

To prevent this sort of theft you need to determine how much of various supplies your practice needs to operate and how much waste is acceptable. For example, if your practice gives 100 allergy shots per month, then you should probably not be spending more than it takes to buy say 105 syringe and needle combinations for this purpose on average. Your need will vary from month to month but you should be able to track about how many of these items will be needed based on your patient volume for that procedure. If you find you're ordering 25 or 50% more setups than you are billing for, then you have a leak that needs to be fixed.

You need to decide what will be the size of the inventory on hand and how much and how often various supplies can be ordered without having to have special approval and explanation for the excess need. Goods that can be used at home (soft drinks, snacks, paper products) are areas where you have to be particularly careful as it's easy for an employee sent to the store to purchase these items from your petty cash supply to just leave some of these supplies in the car when they arrive back at the office. You need a receipt and change for these purchases and they need to be for the quantity you've approved. If the items are used to generate charges (medications, lab draws etc.) Periodically comparing orders to charge counts is a good check of both processes.

Note that printer toner cartridges could be replaced before they're truly empty and taken home for their final thousand pages of use. It's a good idea to make sure expended items like this are really discarded and don't wind up causing you to order more than you should. Printer paper is particularly difficult to track since you can't control how many faxes you will receive for example but keeping track of average use will at least make you aware when usage goes higher than can be explained by variations in how busy the practice is.

Be aware that supplies can also be stolen by diverting deliveries. For example, an employee can (if you let the employees place these orders) ask that some supplies be delivered to some other location than your office from time to time. An alternate location could be their apartment but more likely would be a vacant office suite in your office building or even a suite that's not vacant if the delivery is timed for a day that business is closed. Then it's a simple matter for the employee-thief to walk over and pick up those packages during their lunch break. Employees can mix personal items they would like to steal with business purchases and can just remove those items from the box when the order is delivered to the office.

Postage machines are another opportunity you have to watch as it only takes seconds for an employee to steal postage to mail personal mail using your postage machine. Never allow employees to "buy" or "borrow" postage from the practice postage machine. If you allow this you have yet one more thing you have to constantly audit to verify fraud is not occurring when you are not watching.

Never allow employees to use your credit card machine as an ATM by running their card on your machine and then taking money from your cash drawer or petty cash supply. While on its face, this may seem a harmless convenience, it is just one more way that employees not normally

authorized to touch cash in your practice can get regular

access to it. Nothing good comes from these casual

practices with your practice resources and funds.

Purchasing accounts

Many vendors will allow your practice to purchase various items or services and will bill you for the items or services on a monthly basis. Remember that it is in the interest of these businesses to make it as easy as possible for you and your practice to order more and more things. As a result, these businesses do not necessarily have much interest in vetting those who place the orders. One major office supply retail store you have probably heard of gave our office a purchasing account. They also gave us a store purchase credit card. The credit card isn't like your MasterCard or Visa in that it isn't associated with any one person. The terms of the card agreement say that the business with the account agrees to pay for any charges on the card no matter who presents the card. There is no checking of identification of the card holder, no

requirement that any particular signature be used, no

requirement that any purchase order accompany the card,

and little or no recourse if an employee or random person

off the street uses the card to purchase laptops, stationery,

or school supplies for their kids. This card can be very

convenient but is a very dangerous thing as well. As bad as

this is, the same store recently allowed some of our

employees to order items in person at the store and have

them placed on the company account without requiring

any proof that these employees were in fact our

employees. When asked, the store manager said they

normally wanted to see an employee ID or check stub to

prove the purchasers are employees but this is not much

protection against an employee (or even a former

employee or their family member or friends) from making an unauthorized purchase and again in spite of the managers claim as to his store's policy, in our case no form of identification was requested or required other than the ability to name a business with an account. If you want to steal from a large office supplier (or their purchase account holders,) all you really have to do is go to the counter with your purchases and guess the name of a local business that might have a purchasing account at that store. They'll even help you look up the name if you don't get it quite right. When we learned of these policies, the company said we could not close our account, that they would close it only if it stopped being used. I told the man I could stop using the account but could not control use of the account by random people off the street that understood their purchasing policies and wanted to add things to my bill.

Many vendors have web sites that allow for orders to be placed. Not all of these sites will require or verify that a business officer or owner is the one setting up the online access to your business account. You may well have online ordering accounts for businesses you aren't even aware of that have been set up by your employees or others. As a policy, you should only use online ordering if you know for a fact that the vendor can limit access to the site to people you personally authorize to place orders. This list should be short and monthly statements have to be closely scrutinized to make sure every item bought and paid for was something your business actually uses and that you authorized for purchase. Any time a bill that is due is missing for a given month you have to call the vendor to

get a duplicate statement issued. You should maintain a list

a bills you receive monthly that you can use as a checklist

every month to make sure none go missing as a missing

bill may be intentionally missing to hide nonbusiness

purchases.

Theft of patient information

Theft of patient information is a difficult and important topic. In most practices, almost every employee has access to a wealth of information about your patients. This of course includes their health problems (including sensitive issues such as their general health, sexually transmitted diseases, and more) as well as their financial information including their checking account bank(s), account numbers, bank routing numbers, signatures, social security numbers, health insurance account(s) and numbers, photographic ID's such as driver's license copies, insurance card copies, credit card numbers including expiration dates and security codes, and more. It doesn't take too much imagination to see where this puts both you and your patients at risk of identity theft or even blackmail if an employee wanted to misuse their access to the information. I said this is a tough area as more likely than not it won't be your employee that actually uses the information stolen from your patients. For example, an employee Sally is a medical assistant in your practice that works part-time. She frequently works through lunch as she doesn't get many hours. While there, she gathers up credit card information and sells the numbers online to a third party that pays her $25 for each credit card or debit card number stolen. The card information is never used by Sally directly. The patients will, from time to time, get random charges for air fare to Europe or Asia or Africa. The patient has no idea the card information was stolen by your employee as the cards typically are used with a variety of merchants both in town and on trips and online.

Since your patients aren't sharing notes with each other or with you for that matter they have no idea of the common link to your practice. On the other hand, if someone does find out, they aren't going to know which of your employees did the deed. In fact, more likely than not, they'll accuse the wrong staffer, not Sally. Either way, you are likely to be liable for Sally's fraud. Beyond the financial cost of such a fraud your reputation will suffer.

Depending on how you handle credit cards and debit cards this may be difficult to prevent but you should be aware of this risk. Make sure you have insurance to cover for such losses and do whatever is possible, working with your bank or card merchant account provider, to find ways to protect the patients (customers) from loss of this valuable information.

Another risk regarding patient medical data is that there have been cases where personal injury attorneys have paid "finders fees" to hospital or medical office employees for referral information for patients who may have been "victims" of either injuries from car accidents, medication side effects, or a bad medical outcome that could be construed as malpractice. Employees need to be informed of the seriousness of such offenses. Inform your employees that not only is the practice liable for this sort of employee behavior but that the employee may also be subject to sanctions and penalties from the government and that you will hold them personally and financially responsible through a lawsuit, if necessary, for any losses suffered by the practice as a result of their behavior.

You can try to notice if there's a pattern of your patients winding up involved with more than the expected amount of litigation, particularly if you see the same legal firm involved more often than expected.

Employees can use patient identification and demographic data to apply for credit in the name of patients living or dead (identify theft). You need to have policies that make it clear to employees how much trouble they can get in if they participate in these schemes. Prevention is difficult. In some cases it may be worthwhile to be proactive and inform new patients in their welcome to the practice brochure that you seriously respect their safety and privacy. Make sure they know that if they suspect any issues with diversion of dollars or information that you really want to know about it immediately so you can be sure your office is not a source of trouble to them. Patients alerted like this are more likely to notice funny charges or unusual names filled in on checks they delivered to pay medical bills.

When you have patients who are public figures or VIP's, you should consider sequestering and/or protecting those records from prying eyes when not in use for legitimate purposes. Most EMR (Electronic Medical Record) software can mark a chart as sensitive. This is used to give further protection and auditing of charts that may belong to employees, the Mayor, or a famous (or notorious) rock star. Tabloids have been known to offer cash rewards for hospital or medical office employees that are willing to divulge juicy gossip they can later publish. Either way, you are likely to face embarrassment and major financial and perhaps HIPAA liability should your employees divert your patient's confidential data in this way. Again you need insurance that will cover for these specific losses as well as pay for defending claims against you for this sort of thing; 100% prevention is not possible.

Theft of business information

Outside parties can steal business data from you with your employees' help. Stealing business information can be as simple as divulging which doctors send you the most referrals - something your competition can use to target their marketing efforts. Pharmaceutical representatives can be the most prolific spreaders of "business gossip" between practices. Some "buy" access to doctors that may not otherwise see them if not for the valuable "business intelligence" (AKA gossip) these reps can provide about the activities of their competition in the market. Even if you don't give sensitive information to the reps, your staff may innocently or otherwise give up this information during normal conversation. Even information about when you plan to be out of town on vacation can be valuable to an employee's cousin who happens to be in the breaking and entering business. Employees need to understand what business information is confidential (i.e. your businesses holiday and vacation schedules, staffing pattern, salaries of staff, referral sources, and referral destinations, practice income, vendor relationships etc.) and what information is public (your own marketing efforts). They need to understand that sales representatives are not real friends though many are professionally trained to simulate and behave as friends for business purposes including training on how to get your confidential information to further their business. Employees need to be careful to avoid pseudo-social contact with representatives and other vendors. I call them pseudo-social as the employees (including doctors) may see these as social. Never forget that the representatives are "on the clock" and are working every time you see them and are specifically trained to create the illusion of social time so you are vulnerable both to their pitches and to revealing confidential business information they can use or perhaps trade with your competition for better access to their practices.

Theft of medications

Medical practices frequently store medications on site, typically therapeutic agents and patient samples. Therapeutic agents could include antibiotics, pain medications (including perhaps narcotics), other controlled substances, and emergency medications. For the purposes of this book, however, there are really just a couple of categories to be concerned with, controlled versus uncontrolled medications. Theft or diversion of uncontrolled medications are an issue much like any other medical supply. You pay for these supplies. If an employee steals them you have to pay for them again, and you may run into shortages that disrupt the operation of your practice. Theft or diversion of controlled medications include the same issues you have with uncontrolled medicines but are more complicated because your practice can gain the attention of various law enforcement organizations including the Federal Drug Enforcement Administration (DEA). You are responsible for controlled substances you purchase and are responsible for maintaining their security, for keeping detailed custody records, and for preventing theft and diversion. Employees who are addicted to drugs or who have close family or "friends" who are addicts or dealers can create all sorts of other problems and liabilities and indeed danger to you and your other employees. Drugs can be stolen by just carrying them out the door but in the case of narcotics theft with normal regulatory monitoring, there are two main ways drugs are diverted. One way to steal a drug is that medication that is intended for a patient can be diverted into the body of the thief instead of that of the patient. The patient receives either a reduced dose or perhaps no dose at all (i.e. saline). Another common method is for an employee to "waste" narcotic into their body. Normally a witness is required when unused or left over narcotic is "wasted." However, it is very common in a busy environment for an employee to take medicine to the sink and announce that he or she is wasting medicine, and another employee within ear shot but not actually in the room with the employee "wasting" medicine agrees to sign off as a witness to the waste of the narcotic that, of course, may or may not have been actually wasted down the drain. It is not uncommon for a drug addicted person to take advantage of unsuspecting "friends", coworkers, or even family members to facilitate their theft of their drug of choice.

Case study - drug diversion

A hospital nurse "John" had a back injury and was prescribed narcotic analgesics. He was a charge nurse in the intensive care unit of a trauma center. When his prescriptions ran out, he realized he needed more medicine. Because he was a well educated nurse very familiar with drug storage and regulations, he started giving himself pain medicines that were documented as routed for his patients who had P.R.N. (as needed) orders for pain medication. In some cases, the patients requested and needed medicine that they didn't get, or got in reduced doses, as he stole part or all of their doses. In other cases, the patients never requested or needed the medicine, but he could easily obtain the drug by documenting a request for

pain medicine. He would then pocket the drug and

document it as given to the patient. Other times he would

take advantage of the waste method noted above.

Eventually he found it so easy and successful that he got

more careless and increased his patients "use" of pain

medications and the pharmacy and nursing management

noted that patients that hardly ever needed pain medicine

always needed the maximum ordered amount of as-needed

medicine for 8 hours followed by 16 hours without a need

for pain medicine. Eventually someone suspected the nurse

was the common link. The pharmacy started auditing his

drug cart and posting staff to watch his patients for several

days before and after his shifts. Patients and other

employees were interviewed, and phones were tapped and

recorded as there was suspicion he might be selling drugs to others. Eventually, when they felt they had all the evidence needed, they stopped him leaving through the employee exit with 2-3 syringes full of an injectable narcotic analgesic in his pocket. He was arrested, lost his license, and went to work in some non-medial field. How could this have been prevented? Obviously enforcement of the requirement for real witnesses for wasted medication would help even though this was a minor part of John's theft pattern. Staff need to be reminded that no matter how educated and qualified and senior the staff member is, addiction can hit anyone and lead to criminal behavior, therefore, employees should not trust anyone so much they sign that they witness things they didn't actually witness. Preventing the diversion of medicines intended for patients is more difficult. Unless you require a second staffer to verify all pain medication requests and have another staffer or security guard follow the nurse from patient to the medicine room to the patient and back, it will be difficult to totally prevent this. John was only caught because he was stealing such a large volume of drugs that it stood out. Had he been less "greedy," he might still be stealing those drugs today.

Many practices correctly determine that stocking and dispensing controlled substances is far more trouble and liability than their convenience or income generating potential is worth.

Theft of credit

Most practices (and most homes for that matter) receive unsolicited offers to extend credit or credit cards. Most of these go into the trash of course, but a dishonest employee can fish these offers out of the trash. Employees frequently know enough about their employer or the employer's business to complete an application. It's possible that a credit card could be issued to the employee's home or even to the business addressed attention to that employee, particularly if you don't get the first access to all incoming mail. Once obtained, the employee could run up charges while discarding the bills or even paying the minimum so they could buy thousands of dollars in merchandise or cash advances until eventually the practice is contacted to find out why the bills aren't being paid or your personal or business credit winds up damaged. Credit card fraud is particularly a risk with employees that are soon going to be leaving your employment as they're less likely to worry about consequences or getting caught. An employee can order items and have the items delivered to addresses other than their home (a vacant apartment, for example) to make it harder to tell who actually stole the credit. The solution, of course, is to restrict who has access to incoming mail either to a manager or better yet an owner of the practice so that credit card applications can be shredded and kept away from people who might use them for evil purposes. Having an owner screen and open incoming mail is helpful for preventing other fraud as well and is a good business practice. Access to mailbox keys should be guarded much like you'd guard the keys to your house or car. If you go

on vacation, stop the mail, if you have to, to maintain

control.

Kickbacks / bribes / referrals for sale

Your choices with respect to from whom you buy supplies, with whom you bank, with whom you use for home health care, physical therapy, radiology services, cardiology services, pulmonary services, oxygen, wheelchairs, hospital beds, hospice, and more are very important to many businesses. Most medical practices control the routing of far more money than they'll ever see as income to their practice. A very competitive marketplace exists in the medical vendor area particularly for home healthcare equipment and hospice agencies.

A specialist may order as many as 700 CT scans per year. At about $2,000 each, that comes out to $1,400,000.00 of business for just one study type that is ordered. Most of this money comes from insurance companies including

Medicare and Medicaid programs. When the market is

competitive, the gain or loss of a single referral source is a

really big deal. The money involved may tempt a vendor to

try to buy influence with your employees (and even you)

and may also tempt your employees to sell influence. Your

referrals can be the difference between wealth and

bankruptcy so the temptation is strong. Of course, every

business that depends on you for referral business wants to

influence you and legitimate marketing is all about this.

The problem comes in where the line is crossed between

legal and illegal inducement. A business could offer a cash

finder's fee (or a gift certificate) for every oxygen referral,

for example, a pretty obvious example of Medicare fraud

or violation of anti-kickback laws, but I've seen such

offers before from people and businesses who you think would know better. More subtle ways to illegally buy influence are to hire people for sham jobs such as consultants or part time labor and pay them for the purposes of either reimbursing referrals or hopefully creating a sense of familiarity that leads to extra referrals indirectly. People by their nature like to help their friends, family and acquaintances, but in a medical practice, one of the last things you need is to get unwanted attention from the Inspector General's office because one of your employees wants to do someone a favor. Even if there is no direct economic impact, this behavior hurts your reputation as an honest practice. If the improperly selected referrals are for vendors you pay for services, then you are probably not using the most cost effective vendor available.

When it comes to buying supplies, many vendors are available, and comparing prices is complicated. It's easy for a vendor to charge more and pass on a part of the extra price to the person that places the order. Unless you take time to shop around, you won't know you're not getting the best possible deal. It's best if you don't leave the choice of vendors up to your employees. Not having this responsibility and authority tremendously limits their influence and value to the vendor and reduces the likelihood that the vendor will route some of your money into their pockets to keep their referrals coming. Allowing a staffer and not your manager to control access of sales representatives to your doctors or lunch meetings also invites special favors for whoever the gatekeeper is.

When it comes to home healthcare or hospice or durable medical equipment referrals, I feel it's best to rotate this business around to all the eligible providers for the patient's payor. This way you avoid fraud and the appearance of fraud and will tend to get better service and attention from all the vendors. Once vendors think they have you in their pocket, they naturally put less effort into keeping your business. Vendors that generate lots of complaints either from your staff or the patients can be threatened with being dropped from your rotation or actually dropped if necessary.

Fake vendors & invoices

As mentioned briefly earlier, it is very important to know every company to whom your business writes checks. Many vendor names are not very descriptive. Unless you do the research, you won't easily know which companies are real and which are bogus. Some medical practice employees have opened checking accounts in names of entities that do not really exist and then send invoices for supplies, equipment, equipment repair, services, or even newsletter subscriptions. An unwitting manager might just pay without question or maybe the manager was actually the one creating the fake vendor and sending the fake bills to the practice? Getting fake bills and invoices for magazines, for example, asking you to renew when you never subscribed in the first place is not rare. They intentionally send an invoice that seems like it should be paid as a routine expense when it's really signing up for $400 of OSHA manuals or some other product you never really ordered. For this reason, the practice owner(s) need to pay close attention to bills paid and compare them to a list of verified vendors. When something new comes in, check it out and see if it's legitimate before just sending a check and adding it to the list. Even fake tax bills that look like some of the legitimate tax bills that seem to arrive at seemingly random times during the year can be a method to separate you from your money.

Payroll fraud

Review time sheets and payroll / check stubs in your

accounting software to make sure no one is getting

supplemental income from categories other than hours

worked and that no one is getting overtime or extra

vacation time beyond what is called for in your policy

manual. Be sure to review these randomly and at the end

of the year.

Someone with access to your payroll system can even

manipulate settings to prevent taxes from being withheld

from a paycheck or can find other ways to adjust pay in

ways you do not authorize. An employee could even

present you with a false social security number that would

result in their income not being reported to the IRS. It's

important to verify the identity and citizenship status of people you hire. When you hire someone under illegal circumstances, you can expect to eventually have trouble from the government. Of course, you've already hired a verified criminal who already has experience thwarting the law before he starts working for you.

In a large practice with many employees, it's even possible that a fake employee could be created and not noticed by management or the practice owners. Cases have been reported in the news media recently where an employee left a business, yet his or her paycheck continued for months.

Forgery

Many practices maintain life insurance for key owners whether to help the practice survive the unscheduled death of a co-owner or to guarantee a practice loan. Be careful that you don't leave sufficient information around to allow an employee to change the beneficiary of the policy to someone you don't authorize. Your staff will be more qualified than most to forge your signature. With today's scanner and PDF file editing software, it's easier than ever to send official documents for various purposes that include your real scanned signature. Signature stamps should be using sparingly if at all and should be controlled like cash. Signatures produced by computers are far better than those produced by signature stamps but not every thief is skilled with the computer and some prefer the low tech signature stamp.

People can "forge" your emails as well. Sarah Palin, while running for Vice President, had her personal Yahoo email account hacked. All the hacker had to do was go online to Yahoo and sign in as her and when prompted for a password, click the "forgotten password" link. This led to security questions (such as the name of a pet and mother's maiden name etc.) that were easily available from public sources, and the email password was reset and delivered to the hacker. Email services vary in what they require of someone to get a password. If your ISP (internet service provider) or email provider uses security questions, give fake answers that you can remember as the people that work with you in your office know better than most the true answers to the most likely security questions. This goes for passwords for online banking sites and credit accounts as well as they may allow all sorts of bad things to happen if compromised.

Electronic medical records can be used to produce prescriptions for controlled substances and it's not too difficult to forge a typically barely legible doctor signature on these as well. Even normal paper prescriptions can be taken home and either used or sold to drug abusers. These prescriptions need not be made out to the employee but could be made out to anyone. The pharmacy would fill the prescription provided the person presenting the prescription could show identification. This could be for a friend or family member, for example. To try to prevent prescription fraud, prescription pads need to be kept locked up and only provided to staff when needed and even then only to staff authorized to write prescriptions. Avoid using your prescription pads intended for medications to order non-medication items such as laboratory or radiology studies. Create special forms for these orders that would not be mistaken for a prescription that might be used for a medication. Check out your EMR/EHR software to make sure electronic prescribing and paper prescribing are appropriately limited and tracked and able to be audited.

Stealing time

Time clock fraud is very common. Employees can arrive late and have their buddy clock them in or can leave early and again have a buddy clock them out. Employees can "forget" to clock in or out and turn in exception sheets to cover early or late departures or arrivals or can "work through lunch" without actually working through lunch. Employees you allow to work from home or outside of normal business hours can drop by to clock in, shop all day, and return later to clock out. Some computer-based time clocks can have their clocks manipulated. Better software that gets its time standard via the internet, not locally, protects against manipulation. If you suspect time clock irregularity, or even if you don't, it may be a good idea to periodically review computer generated logs of activity. Most billing systems have audit logs. Many, if not turned on by default, can be turned on to show the date and time that any chart is accessed. To do billing or medical record work without frequently accessing the system is impossible; a log that shows hours of no activity with the employee on the clock is good evidence of theft of time. Clinical staff also need to access the computer to see the schedule and to deal with charts and EMR/EHR software usually also has a log and/or audit feature that can be used to reconstruct how employees spend their time. Another option is the use of key logging software that records activity including keys pressed and mouse clicks. Many programs can email screen images periodically or when certain keywords are typed. This software can show everything typed, every program run, every website visited, every IM or text message or email sent and every

password entered. Don't forget key logging can be used

against you to get your passwords and confidential banking

information as well if you give sufficient access to your

computer.

Captain of the ship

The captain of the ship is traditionally responsible for what happens on his or her command. Fraudulent or illegal activity on the part of your employees at one level or another could create liability for you and your practice. An employee could incorrectly code your visits to a level higher than justified by the medical facts, hoping to impress you with their ability to bring in more money. In some cases, this could result in your being banned from Medicare or other insurer participation and could cause you to be liable for a fine or refund based on a small statistical sample showing the error. Improper release of protected medical information to the media or elsewhere could cause you to be charged with a violation HIPAA (privacy laws) and subject you to liability that may not be covered by your insurer (read the policies to see). A staffer's failure to deliver a test result to a patient could cause a delay in a cancer diagnosis or a failure to get a test scheduled in a timely fashion could cause a heart attack to not be prevented. All of these can create liability. Proper documentation of unsuccessful attempts to contact a patient about important health matters can be the difference between being liable or not. Obviously, no one can prevent all the ways an employee can get you in trouble, and you certainly cannot be in business without employees that you can trust and rely on. Most employees try to do their best for you, but it is important that you understand the risks of working with employees and are alert to clues of problems to come. If you can understand and recognize your vulnerabilities, you can at least try to mitigate the risks and recover from human caused

disasters. Check with your insurer too to make sure you

have not only malpractice policies but general liability and

acts and omissions policy coverage.

Entrapment & workplace injury fraud

Another ugly but real problem is that an employee can come to work with you with plans to become disabled due to a workplace incident or injury that is either faked or exaggerated for the purpose of obtaining perhaps life long disability payments and other insurance benefits. He/she can also try to make a personal injury lawsuit out of the incident and sue you and the practice for damages. You should have insurance to cover for as many eventualities as you can afford. Consider having insurance that covers for acts and omissions, medical malpractice, general and umbrella liability coverage, employment practices insurance (including coverage for discrimination claims, sexual harassment claims, labor law violation claims and so on), and coverage for any other risk you or your attorney may feel is an issue in your state of practice.

While you cannot easily protect against false claims, you can reduce the risk by avoiding practices that expose you to excess liability. Risky practices include: serving or allowing the use of alcohol at business lunches or parties, having social relationships with employees or their family members, providing special benefits for anyone as those not getting the benefits will assume the worst even if all is innocent.

If you are careful and document well, you may well win most suits brought against you. Unfortunately, if a suit is brought against you, you've already lost because of the time, expense, and emotional toll of defending a suit even if, and maybe especially, if not legitimate. Clearly your best response is to do what you can to avoid the suit in the first place. Make it clear that you are careful and defend any lawsuits as strongly as possible. Ask your lawyer about things you can do to bring consequences to anyone who sues you unsuccessfully with false allegations.

Credit cards / debit cards

These days it is difficult to do business without a credit or debit card. Cards are needed for business travel and for business purchases either at stores or online. The actual credit card should always be controlled by one or more owners of the practice. In a medical group, it should be clear what purposes the card or cards can and will be used for. Your accountant can explain the difference between business (deductible) and nonbusiness expenses for which you can legitimately use practice cards. At times, an employee or your office manager will need to order something online or to pay for a repair or service call where a credit card may be useful. However, handing your practice card or card numbers over to anyone basically invites him/her at some time in the future to steal from you in case of "emergency". An employee could hold on to that number for months or years without using it, but, when under pressure, he may use the card, long after you have forgotten the circumstances where you gave up the numbers. For those cases where something needs to be ordered with a card, you can either do the transaction yourself rather than sharing the number, or you can get a disposable one-time number issued by the bank for this purpose. These card numbers are available from PayPal, American Express, Citibank and many others. You get the card issuer to issue you a disposable one-time use credit card number that links to your account. You can frequently generate these yourself with a few clicks online with the bank's website. You give the disposable number to your employee or manager who needs to order something for the practice; once used, this number is cancelled with no more access to your credit card account for future purchases. If you have a practice debit card, always answer CREDIT when the vendor or store asks you DEBIT or CREDIT. You get protections when using these cards as CREDIT that you do not have when you use them as DEBIT cards. If there is fraudulent use or identify theft, you will have an easier time getting restitution from the card issuer if the card is used as a CREDIT card.

You may be able to get your bank to mail a duplicate credit card and checking account statement to your home so you can make sure statements that go missing or that may be missing pages at the office don't hide shady transactions from your attention.

Checking accounts

Every practice has a checking account. If you have two or more owners, then ask for a two signature requirement for checks. This requirement keeps partners honest and keeps them informed what money is being spent on what. Two sets of eyes are better than one when it comes to spotting irregularities. Insist that when your manager prepares bills to be paid, that checks presented for signing are always given to you with the invoices/bills/statements attached, so you never sign a check without looking at the statement and understanding what is being paid for. First verify that the vendor is legitimate. Next, ask for explanations if the total bill looks unusual or if there are items listed on the invoice that are out of the ordinary or in out of the ordinary quantity.

Avoid using online bill paying services with your business account or allowing Quicken or Quickbooks type office financial or accounting software to electronically pay your bills. Though great, cost effective, and convenient products when used to handle your home finances, you don't want to use any system that allows an employee or even your accountant to write electronic payments to a hotel in Tahiti while bypassing your signature requirement with the bank.

You should look at your checking account statements on a regular basis and should balance your checkbook from time to time rather than leaving this to a manager. A corrupt manager could write a check for a personal item using your business checking account and could cover this by changing the checkbook entry to something that looks more legitimate like a payment to a valid vendor. Unless you compare checks returned from the bank to your check ledger entry you could miss this. To use this method, your employee would need to be able to sign the check for you but forgery and signatures stamps aren't rare so beware.

Avoid giving anyone electronic access to your account. If a loan or lease deal gives you a better deal or makes a loan contingent on ACH transfers from your account, just open up a new account especially for that purpose and fund it every month. Never add to the list of people with access to take money from your account. Even if they aren't stealing from you, it is difficult to win a dispute with someone who can draft disputed payments from you automatically.

Tell the bank in writing that no one is authorized to give telephone authority for a wire transfer from your account. One bank I used to bank with allowed a former employee (who was later arrested) to phone in a wire transfer to pay a personal bill. That employee was not authorized to sign checks and had no official capacity at all with respect to the bank, but over the years became known to one of the tellers we frequently dealt with so the teller just assumed the wire must be authorized. Sure this is banking malpractice, but I think it's good practice to put the bank on written notice that no one is authorized to do wire transfers so the bank has no place to hide in the event they process a payment you did not authorize.

Part III - Billing related theft & fraud

Overview of cash flow

This is arguably the most important process that must be secured to avoid theft on a scale that can easily threaten the solvency of your practice. Practices that lose $100,000 or more usually lose it in this area. Most medical practices collect hundreds of dollars per day, per provider, across the counter at patient check-in or check-out. The money consists of cash, credit card payments, checks, and money orders. Additional money is typically mailed to the practice in checks large and small from patients and from medical insurance companies, as well as from other practices that may purchase professional services from you (such as interpretation fees for x-rays, EKG's, echocardiograms, ultrasounds, or other items). Checks are also sent from lawyers for professional consultations, worker's

compensation evaluations, and medical records requests in

support of disability applications among other things.

Billing fraud is a complex topic with many risks and

opportunities for conversion of your money into money in

the pocket of thieves.

Let's review the flow of cash through your practice. The

typical workflow for an office visit is:

-the patient makes an appointment;

-when the patient arrives a router or ticket is created to

keep up with the charges for this visit;

-You mark the patient as arrived in the computer;

-the computer or the patient's insurance card says a co-payment (say $40) is needed. The money is typically contractually required to be paid at the time the patient checks in (before seeing the doctor);

-the amount paid is normally written on the router;

-at some point, the payment is entered into the billing computer system to reflect a $40 credit to the patients account to be applied to the final bill for that visit when it's available;

-the patient then gets seen by the provider;

-typically the charges generated during the visit are written onto the router or ticket;

-at some point, maybe today or maybe tomorrow those charges are entered into the computer;

-a bill is generated and transmitted, usually electronically, to the insurance company who will likely eventually pay some portion of the bill and adjust off some portion of the bill;

-any remaining patient responsibility balance is then billed to the patient and may be paid via the mail or collected at the window at a future office visit;

-the money collected for a given day is typically stored in a box and eventually taken to the bank for a deposit.

Because the bank deposit may not happen every day the practice is open (indeed the practice could be open days the bank is closed or could be open later than the bank), correlating bank deposits with the date the money was actually received in the office is often not easy. Money deposited will not only include money given to the practice on the same day as a visit for that day's charges, but will also include any payments across the counter for services delivered but not yet paid for from previous dates. The deposit may also include money mailed to the practice by patients for multiple dates of service or from insurers or other parties (see above) for various dates of service. This creates some complexity when you produce a computer report to try to determine the amount of a day's deposit to reconcile with a bank statement particularly since deposits for multiple days of business may be delivered to the bank at once to create a few large deposits per week.

Remember that cash is your most vulnerable commodity because it's so negotiable. When a patient delivers cash to a practice either to settle an old bill or to purchase something from your practice or to pay a co-payment, the cash that is delivered is instantly negotiable by anyone. Once in a pile there's no easy way to say from whom the money came and to where it should go, and no one has to prove he is anyone in particular to be able to use that cash.

Here are some methods an employee can use to steal cash from your practice. I will also discuss measures you can take to either prevent the method from being used or to detect the crime when it happens. Note that some practices such as having an owner collect mail from the mailbox every day to remove payments or stamping FOR DEPOSIT ONLY on all checks immediately as they are received can help prevent a variety of schemes to steal your money.

Lose the router

This is one of the worst methods of theft for the practice. The check-in person collects the co-payment, pockets the cash, and shreds the router. Not only are you missing the co-payment, you're not even entering a bill for all the services delivered the day of the visit. No claim goes to the insurer and no bill goes to the patient. The employee gets $40, and you might lose $500 from the encounter. Patients sometimes steal routers to prevent charges from being entered as well - particularly when they know their insurance information is bogus or they are self-pay patients. Prevention is that routers have to be treated like you treat checks in your personal checkbook. They have to be numbered, tracked, and accounted for every day. A missing router is evidence of fraud until proven otherwise.

Employees need to understand this relationship and realize if they're careless and lose a router that they will need to defend themselves.

Every dollar collected from a patient must generate a receipt with a copy to the patient and a copy to the practice. Use a receipt book with "carbon copy" numbered receipts in a book format, so you can tell if one is missing and can quickly see a copy of every receipt written. The administrator (or better yet an owner) must review all routers every day to verify there is a match for every appointment for the date with all no shows and cancellations accounted for and verified. The co-payment or other payment recorded on the router must match the receipt book and match the money box and match the deposit every day. Indeed this needs to be checked every day without fail. It should be obvious that the person doing these checks should not be the person who actually collects the money and delivers the receipts and prepares the deposit slip. This is one of the most important areas where the sin of "concentration" is not allowed.

The charges on the router must be entered into the billing system as soon as possible after the visit as well as posting to the patient account any money paid at the time of the visit. All of these need to match up with the deposit batch from counter collections. The verifying and auditing cannot be valid if the same person collecting the money is the one verifying the accounting of the money. Ideally, you should bundle all counter collected funds into a separate deposit slip for a separate deposit to the bank for each day you are open. Even if you only go to the bank every four days, on that day you go to the bank, you should carry at least four separate deposits, one for each day you are open, that include only the money collected over the counter. This makes it easy to use your billing system to generate a report that will match the deposit slip and the actual deposit to the bank with the total of the receipts written for that date. Other deposited money such as that money delivered by way of the mail can go in its own batch and deposit slip and should be reconciled with money posted to accounts that was not collected across the counter.

Short the deposit

Another method of billing theft is an employee can pocket the cash portion of a payment (or just part of it) and can give the patient full credit for the payment in the billing system (to prevent them getting billed for what was stolen) and just have the deposit come up short, taking advantage of the fact that it is difficult to reconcile the deposits with daily collections since they come from so many sources. The answer to this problem and many other methods of theft of cash is that deposits to the bank need to be separated by their source. The deposits for money collected across the counter should never combine more than one office day and should not be blended with deposits from other sources such as insurance checks or bills paid from patients through the mail. If one person works check-in/check-out in the morning and another the afternoon, you should consider making two separate deposits or even using two separate locked cash boxes with each box assigned to the person who will be held responsible for the contents of the box at the end of the day. If more than one employee has access to the cash box during a day, then responsibility for the contents belongs to both and neither, a perfect opportunity for theft that you can't easily pin on the individual who is responsible. Stores and restaurants typically audit the cash drawer when cashiers change even if just for a break. This way there is accountability for the contents of the deposit.

Case study - go ask Alice

Alice was an office manager that took care to make sure and reconcile router information with deposit amounts prepared by Jane, the check-in person. Alice actually caught Jane diverting funds to her own pocket using the Lost Router method described previously. Further investigation (and a patient complaint) also showed Jane had filled her own name in on a patient's check made out to no one. The patient actually asked who was this Jane who had cashed her check.

One day, Alice learned she could take the deposit slip prepared by the Jane and rewrite the deposit slip minus half the cash before taking the deposit to the bank. She knew the daily deposit contained money collected a variety of ways and that it would be difficult if not impossible for anyone to reconcile deposits with collections given the mixture of sources of deposited money. Alice was eventually caught when one of the doctors noted it had been awhile since anyone had seen the practice credit card bill. Once a copy of the bill was obtained from the bank, it was obvious that many internet store orders for clothing items were being delivered to Alice's home. Once this one statement was examined, all the statements for the prior two years were obtained and audited revealing thousands of dollars of theft over a period of two years. Alice had been employed by the practice for about ten years. This discovery prompted a general audit. Other methods of theft were also discovered and documented. The police were called; Alice was arrested and provided a written confession. Against the objections of the victims, the police insisted Alice be allowed into a pre trial intervention program (PTI) since these were only her first fifty offenses of theft from an employer, and they didn't think the case was important enough for jail time. The police actually threatened to drop all charges if the practice continued to object to their plans for PTI. Alice was fired but within weeks was working in the billing department of another practice. Great news for them.

Alice had worked for the practice for many years and really had never worked anywhere else. She was entrusted with supervising other staff and indeed had caught another employee stealing, yet just because she was a long time employee and a manager did not mean she could be trusted to deal with money headed to the bank. No matter how much you pay a manager or how much you think you trust her, you cannot really feel safe unless you take the cash issue out of their hands and personally, as the business owner, get involved and stay involved daily in supervising cash flowing through your practice. Constant supervision, is time consuming and very inconvenient and may cause some employees to think you don't trust them, but unfortunately it's necessary. You cannot afford to trust staffers not only with your income but with the survival of your entire business and the jobs of all your employees. It's a rare employee you can trust implicitly with so much at stake; even for the one you can really trust, circumstances can change due to debt, lost jobs, illness, divorce, addictions, pressure or threats from family members or friends, etc. Today's trusted employee can

easily become tomorrow's thief.

Adjustments

A billing system savvy check-in/check-out person or medical biller can pocket all or part of a cash payment to the practice by just adding an adjustment to offset that part of the debt from the patient's account. This effectively reduces the patient's bill by the amount that was stolen, so the patient is not billed for the money he has already paid. This is difficult to detect unless you happen to look at that patient's account and see an adjustment that can't be explained otherwise.

Adjustments are a common way an employee might give a "discount" to a friend or family member who happens to be a patient of the practice. This method could even be used to waive the contractually required co-payment you

144

have to collect from patients before they are seen. This theft from the employer is bad enough. The insurer or Medicare, however, will see this as insurance or Medicare fraud. Even though the employee is clearly the criminal, the employer is the one with the contractual and legal obligation to collect the co-payments and could face additional liability for the actions of the employee giving their buddy a $40 discount on an office visit. Losing a router or just failing to enter all the charges associated with an encounter is another way an employee might give a patient a discount you have not authorized. However, if you use the method noted above of recording all patient payments on the router and then reconciling the total of the money on the routers with the deposit and the receipt book, you will prevent many fraudulent transactions at check-in/

check-out. Theft, however, is more difficult to detect if done by the medical biller dealing with cash paid to the practice at times other than a visit when the patient is not present, and no router is generated to be tracked. To prevent theft of this cash, you are better off making sure that cash and checks, for that matter, are never mailed to the practice. This is accomplished by using a Lockbox and by taking advantage of insurers who are able to wire transfer their payments directly to your practice checking account rather than mailing you a check.

Refunds

Patients with credits on their accounts typically have checks written to them from the practice either periodically or upon request. A dishonest medical biller can create fake patient accounts that generate a need for refunds and can then have checks issued to refund to these fake patients (who may in fact be friends or relatives of the biller that may or may not have been patients of the practice). One method is to allow the family member to receive a medical service from the practice, bill the insurance and patient, and after payment is received, adjust some of the charges creating a refund that is then issued to the patient. Prevention of fraudulent refunds comes from paying extra attention to accounts belonging to friends of relatives of your office manager or medical biller or others with access to and knowledge of how to manipulate the billing system.

A good practice is to randomly review samples of accounts

periodically to verify that charges, payments, and

adjustments are indeed legitimately entered and directed

by the insurer's Explanation of Benefits (EOB's) and not

the whims of a criminally inclined staffer.

Check diversion

Checks, as well as cash, can be stolen from your practice. It is common for checks to be given to the practice with the "Pay to the Order of" line blank. Patients do this to save time, knowing you have a rubber stamp with the practice name you can stamp onto the check. This blank invites a dishonest employee to just write their own name on the check and take and deposit or cash the check. This dishonesty works better for him if he uses a name other than his own for which he can produce acceptable identification, or if he deposits it into another account he controls that doesn't point immediately back to them such as the account of a friend or relative with a different name. Many people do not get their checks returned with their bank statements, and many don't look at each check very carefully. For this method to work, the employee has to use one of the other methods already detailed to hide the theft such as losing the router or adjusting off the payment or just posting the payment if he knows no one is reconciling the router with the deposit and the receipts and appointments. I suggest that you make your staff aware of a policy to refuse any checks delivered blank - post a sign with a brief way to name the practice (perhaps initials or a short version of the practice name) that the bank approves and require the patient to fill out the check completely. You have to audit and reconcile every day as described previously to make sure no routers are missing and that what was collected was really deposited. Checks received by the practice whether across the counter or in the mail should be immediately stamped with a "For Deposit Only" in the name of the practice rather than waiting until the

deposit is prepared at the end of the day. Checks stamped

this way are more difficult to divert. You could even

consider making it policy that the check-in person will

make a point to show this process of stamping the back of

the check to the patient at the time of check-in. Your

patients will see and get used to the practice and are more

likely to be suspicious of a change in behavior. The

employee is also reminded that people are watching his or

her process with respect to handling incoming checks.

Another way to steal checks routed to the practice is to

open a bank account at an alternate bank with a name close

enough to the practice name that they will allow the

deposit and/or cashing of checks made out to your

practice. Banks are not nearly security conscious enough to make this very difficult. I opened a bank account this week in the name of my business, and while I had to show my own ID and produce a tax id number (which is not difficult for any employee or vendor for that matter to find,) I did not have to prove I owned or even worked at the practice. I was able the next day to deposit a check made out to my practice with no questions asked. If I can do this, I'm sure an employee can do it. Someone not planning to be around for long in a busy practice could conceivably save up thousands of dollars of insurance payments (if a Lockbox isn't being used - see above) and walk out one day, deposit the money, and move to Canada with your insurance payments. Many banks do not scrutinize deposited checks enough to even notice that a check is not made out to the person making the deposit. This is particularly true if the deposit is made via a night deposit box or automated teller machine since the customer is not around to show identification or answer questions about the fraudulent deposit.

A particularly tricky way to divert income to an employee is for the employee to replace the practice's deposit slips with nearly identical deposit slips that cause money to be deposited into an account you don't control. The bank will scan the account number and may well not pay much attention to the fact that the account number and account name don't match, but even if they did look, the thief's account could have a name similar enough to escape notice.

An incoming insurance check can be redirected to an employee's bank similarly with the account kept as unpaid in the billing system. Invariably there will be accounts that are slow to be paid or that are never paid by an insurance company for one reason or another. A missing insurance payment here or there could easily be missed provided they aren't excessive. As an owner, here is an example of where it's worth your time to really learn how to use your billing system and how to read EOB's and how to track an unpaid account. To catch this method, you eventually have to become suspicious enough that you either find the EOB or get a reprint from the insurer to show that the insurer indeed paid the practice. Maybe someone just forgot to credit the patient account with the payment, or maybe that check is paying for someone's boat. To be sure, you can get the insurer to produce a copy of the cashed check to see into what account it went when cashed.

Some checks arrive to practices that are not expected. Payments for medical records or form completions frequently arrive with the record request and are typically never recorded as bills, and no router is created. These are easy to steal since they aren't expected and will not be missed. While the amounts are typically small, you may want to think about methods to track these small unexpected checks so there is accountability. Again a key here is controlling incoming mail with money removed before the mail goes anywhere else.

Conclusion

By now you should know that no practice is safe from employee theft and that the vast majority of practices have already been victims of employee theft. You now understand many of the ways employees can steal from a practice and why the practice is so attractive and in fact frequently easy to accomplish. You are aware you may not get much help from police after the fact and know that most practice owners have little or no training or experience in accounting for money in the business setting.

It is to be hoped that by understanding the methods commonly used to steal money from medical practices, you know better what to look for and how to close holes in your security and accounting methods to both deter and detect theft by employees.

You understand that no methods to protect your practice can be 100% effective, and that just as important as deterrence and detection is to prepare for losses when they come. Preparation for loss means you know what you have, have properly insured against losses for which you can insure, and have backup copies of important papers and computer data that you can't replace with money alone.

This field is constantly changing as laws change, insurance regulations and practices change, and employees and others with criminal intent come up with new methods to steal from medical practices. If you have been a victim of employee theft, and particularly if methods were used that

have not been described in this book, I would appreciate

your sending an email so your examples could possibly be

used in a future edition of the book.

Send your contributions to me at StealFromDoc@me.com.

Resources

The following links can provide additional information about best practices to avoid and how to detect medical office employee theft.

StealFromDoc.com

http://www.StealFromDoc.com

This site is set up to support readers of this book. The site has excerpts from the text, breaking news articles, and a forum where readers can contribute their own ideas about methods of embezzlement and prevention of embezzlement from medical practices.

The Association of Certified Fraud Examiners

http://www.acfe.com/

Many articles on various sources of fraud and how to investigate and prevent. Not specific to medical practices but many principles apply to all businesses subject to theft.

Averti Fraud Solutions

http://www.avertifraudsolutions.com/

A company that provides online articles and consulting services to help fight fraud in the office environment with particular attention to medical practice fraud and theft.

Medical Group Management Association

http://www.mgma.com

This site has many resources to assist with managing a

medical group. Not limited to information about fraud and employee theft, though there are certainly articles on this topic as well as other general medical group management information.

Practice Support Resources, Inc.

http://www.practicesupport.com/

Variety of texts and manuals on various aspects of medical practice management.

Spector Soft

http://www.spectorsoft.com

Key logging/computer monitoring software for Mac OS and Windows.

About the author

Dr. Donald Elton lives in Columbia, SC. He completed his

undergraduate education with an associate in science in

Respiratory Care from Midlands Technical College in

Columbia, SC, and a bachelor of science degree in biology

from the University of South Carolina in Columbia, SC.

He completed medical school at the Medical University of

South Carolina in Charleston, SC, and completed his

internal medicine residency and pulmonary diseases

fellowship at the University of South Carolina / Dorn

Veterans Hospital / Palmetto Health Richland Hospitals in

Columbia, SC. He has practiced pulmonary and critical

care medicine in Orlando, FL, and Columbia, SC, and has

practiced emergency medicine in Orlando, FL and Sumter,

SC. He has two children and is an instrument rated private

pilot. His medical interests include pulmonary vascular diseases, left ventricular diastolic dysfunction, clinical research, and education.

Dr. Elton can be reached by email at:

StealFromDoc@me.com

His practice website is:

http://LexingtonPulmonary.com

You can also follow the Twitter feed at:

http://www.twitter.com/StealFromDoc

The book has a supporting website including a forum for

reader discussion at:

http://www.StealFromDoc.com